The Ketogenic Guide For Beginners

Adriana S. Brotherton

Contents

1. Introduction 1
2. Tacos de Pork 5
3. Lamb Chops from Italy 9
4. Stir-fried pork 13
5. Meatballs 17
6. Pork Tenderloin Made Simple 21
7. Poultry Chicken Avocado Salad 23
8. Chicken with Paprika 25
9. Chicken Parmesan 29
10. Chicken Wings 33
11. Chicken with Lemon 37
12. Delicious Chicken Skewers 41
13. Delicious Shredded Chicken 43
14. Yogurt Chicken 45
15. Salad with Chicken Bacon 47

16. Mahi Mahi grilled 49
17. Salad with Crab 53
18. Shrimp with Garlic 57
19. Salad de poisson facile 61
20. Crab Cakes Made Simple 65
21. Cod in Butter 69
22. Tilapia Bake 73
23. Avocado Salad with Shrimp 77
24. Shrimp with Paprika 81
25. Soups and Side Dishes 83
26. Soup with Celery 87
27. Soup with Cauliflower Flavor 91
28. Zucchini Basil Soup 95
29. Chicken Soup, Warm and Delicious 99
30. Soup with Creamy Mushrooms 103
31. Soup with Kale and Cauliflower 107
32. Pumpkin Soup 111
33. Cauliflower Soup with Chicken 113
34. Cauliflower Soup with Chicken 117

35. Desserts 121
36. Fat Bombs Chocó 123
37. Frosty Chocolate Delight 125
38. Mousse de strawberries 127
39. Mousse Cheesecake 129
40. Dessert with berries and cheese 131
41. Fudge with Chocó Peanut Butter 133
42. Fat Bombs with Raspberry 135
43. Lemon Mug Cake in a Hurry 137
44. Tiramisu Mousse, Smooth and Silky 139
45. Conclusion 141

Chapter One

Introduction

People in today's society are becoming increasingly health concerned and are looking for ways to keep their weight in a healthy range. The majority of individuals currently confront a problem with their health as a direct result of the rise in pollution levels. These problems include stress, obesity, and hypertension. These health problems are a direct result of the bad eating habits that are being practised.

The ketogenic diet was widely employed during this time period (the 1920s and 1930s) for the treatment of epilepsy. It is also utilised in the treatment of people who suffer from cancer, as keto stops cancer cells from utilising glucose as a source of energy. It stops the proliferation of cells and starves cancer cells, which kills them. Recent studies and research provide evidence that the ketogenic diet can successfully treat a variety of illnesses, including Alzheimer's disease,

Parkinson's disease, epilepsy, metabolic syndrome, obesity, and high blood pressure. Patients with type 2 diabetes also benefit from the keto diet's ability to help them maintain a healthy blood sugar level.

The keto diet is more than simply an eating plan; it's also a way of life and one of the healthier eating habits. The keto diet is particularly helpful for producing quick weight loss. Glucose is the primary fuel source for our body when it is functioning normally. Foods low in carbohydrates are required to be consumed while following the ketogenic diet. It will lower the amount of glucose that is absorbed into your body. Instead of using glucose as fuel, your body uses the fat stores it has.

This book will walk you through the steps of adopting a keto diet after the age of 50 and will explain the many benefits of doing so for your health. My intention is to present you with any and all information that is pertinent to the keto diet after the age of 50. After reading this book, you should have a good understanding of the ketogenic diet, including what foods to consume and which ones to avoid.

Lamb Chops Grilled

Time to prepare: 10 minutes

Time to prepare: 10 minutes

Serve: 6

Ingredients:

Lamb chops, 2 pounds

14 cup extra virgin olive oil

1 teaspoon lemon zest

12 teaspoon pepper

1 tablespoon chopped fresh rosemary

1 tablespoon minced garlic

14 teaspoon kosher salt Instructions:

1.

Combine the garlic, oil, lemon zest, rosemary, pepper, and salt in a mixing bowl.

2.

Place the lamb chops in a bowl with the marinade and let aside to marinate for 1 hour.

3.

Preheat the grill to medium-high.

4.

Sear marinated lamb chops for 2-3 minutes on each side on a hot grill.

5.

Cook for 5-6 minutes over medium heat, or until internal temperature reaches 150 F.

6.

Serve and have fun.

Nutritional Value (Serving Size):

358 calories

Fat 19.6 g

0.9 g carbohydrates

Sugar 0 g

42.6 g protein

136 mg cholesterol

Chapter Two

Tacos de Pork

Time to prepare: 10 minutes

8-hour cooking time

Serve: 8

Ingredients:

pork tenderloin, 2 pounds

23.5 oz salsa

2 1/2 teaspoon powdered garlic

1 1/2 tbsp cumin powder

2 tablespoons chilli powder

1 1/2 teaspoon cayenne

1 1/2 teaspoon salt Instructions:

1.

In a slow cooker, place the meat.

2.

Combine all remaining ingredients (excluding salsa) in a small bowl.

3.

Rub the meat with the spice mixture. Pour the salsa over the pork.

4.

Cook on low for 8 hours with the lid on the slow cooker.

5.

Take the meat out of the slow cooker and shred it with a fork.

6.

Stir the shredded meat back into the slow cooker.

7.

Serve and have fun.

Nutritional Value (Serving Size):

201 calories

Fat 4 g

7.5 g carbohydrates

Sugar 3 g

30 g protein

83 mg cholesterol

Chapter Three

Lamb Chops from Italy

Time to prepare: 10 minutes

15 minutes to prepare

Serve: 4

Ingredients:

Lamb chops, 8

2 tablespoons olive oil

2 tablespoons mustard

1/2 teaspoon of Italian seasoning

1 teaspoon minced garlic

Pepper

Salt

Directions:

1.

Preheat the oven to 425 degrees Fahrenheit.

2.

Place pork chops on a baking pan and season with pepper and salt.

3.

Combine the other ingredients in a small bowl and ladle over each pork chop, spreading evenly.

4.

15 minutes in the oven

5.

Serve and have fun.

Nutritional Value (Serving Size):

391 calories

Fat 21.2 g

1 g carbohydrate

Sugar 0.5 g

48 g protein

150 mg cholesterol

Chapter Four

Stir-fried pork

Time to prepare: 10 minutes

15 minutes to prepare

Serve: 4

Ingredients:

1 pound pork ground

1/2 teaspoon chilli sauce

1 tbsp low-sodium soy sauce

3 minced garlic cloves

1/2 cup chopped cilantro

1/4 cup chopped green onion

2 chopped jalapeo peppers

1 tablespoon lemon juice

1 tablespoon minced ginger

2 tablespoons sesame oil

1 tablespoon extra virgin olive oil

1.

In a medium-sized skillet, heat the oil.

2.

Sauté for a minute with the garlic and ginger.

3.

Cook until the pork is browned.

4.

When the meat is done, whisk in the remaining ingredients thoroughly.

5.

Serve and have fun.

Nutritional Value (Serving Size):

415 calories

Fat 31 g

3 g carbohydrates

Sugar 1 g

20 g protein

121 mg cholesterol

Chapter Five

Meatballs

Time to prepare: 10 minutes

Time to prepare: 20 minutes

Serve: 12

Ingredients:

1 egg

1 pound of ground beef

1 pound ground pork

a half teaspoon of garlic powder

2 tablespoons chopped onion

coconut milk, 1/3 cup

1/4 cup shredded parmesan cheese

1/4 cup chopped fresh parsley

1 tablespoon of Italian seasoning

1 tablespoon almond flour

Pepper

Salt

Directions:

1.

Preheat the oven to 400 degrees Fahrenheit.

2.

In a large mixing basin, combine all of the ingredients and stir thoroughly.

3.

Place the meat mixture in tiny balls on a baking dish.

4.

20 minutes in the oven

5.

Serve and have fun.

Nutritional Value (Serving Size):

192 calories

Fat 7 g

4 g carbohydrates

Sugar 0.7 g

24 g protein

80 mg cholesterol

Chapter Six

Pork Tenderloin Made Simple

Time to prepare: 10 minutes

30 minutes to prepare

Serve: 6

Ingredients:

2 pound pork tenderloin rub

1 tablespoon onion powder 1 tablespoon garlic powder

1 tablespoon of paprika

1/2 teaspoon salt Instructions:

1.

Preheat the oven to 425 degrees Fahrenheit.

2.

Combine all rub ingredients in a small bowl and rub over pork.

3.

Cook over medium-high heat, spraying the pan with cooking spray.

4.

Sear the pork until it is softly golden brown on all sides.

5.

Roast for approximately 25-30 minutes in a preheated oven.

6.

Cut and serve.

Nutritional Value (Serving Size):

228 calories

Fat 5.5 g

2.6 g carbohydrates

Sugar 0.9 g

40.1 g protein

110 mg cholesterol

Chapter Seven

Poultry Chicken Avocado Salad

Time to prepare: 10 minutes

Time to prepare: 10 minutes

Serve: 3

Ingredients:

2 cooked and diced chicken breasts

1 tablespoon lime juice

2 peeled and pitted avocados

2 chopped Serrano chilli peppers

1/4 cup chopped celery

1 chopped onion

1 cup chopped cilantro

1 teaspoon of kosher salt

1.

Using a spoon, scoop out the avocado flesh and set it in the bowl.

2.

Using a fork, mash the avocado flesh.

3.

Mix in the other ingredients until completely blended.

4.

Serve and have fun.

Nutritional Value (Serving Size):

236 calories

Fat 10.6 g

4.5 g carbohydrates

Sugar 1 g

29 g protein

87 mg cholesterol

Chapter Eight

Chicken with Paprika

Time to prepare: 10 minutes

35-minute cooking time

Serve: 4

Ingredients:

4 skinless, boneless chicken breasts, cut into pieces

2 tablespoons paprika

2 1/2 tablespoons extra virgin olive oil

1 1/2 teaspoon minced garlic

2 tablespoons lemon juice

Pepper

Salt

Directions:

1.

Preheat the oven to 350 degrees Fahrenheit.

2.

Combine garlic, lemon juice, paprika, and olive oil in a small bowl.

3.

Season the chicken with salt and pepper.

4.

Pour 1/3 of the bowl mixture into the casserole dish's bottom.

5.

Rub the dish sauce over the chicken in the casserole dish.

6.

Rub the leftover sauce all over the chicken.

7.

30–35 minutes in the oven

8.

Serve and have fun.

Nutritional Value (Serving Size):

380 calories

Fat 22 g

2.6 g carbohydrates

Sugar 0.5 g

43 g protein

130 mg cholesterol

Chapter Nine

Chicken Parmesan

Time to prepare: 10 minutes

35-minute cooking time

Serve: 4

Ingredients:

1 pound skinless and boneless chicken breasts

1/2 cup grated parmesan cheese

mayonnaise, 3/4 cup

1 teaspoon powdered garlic

1/2 teaspoon of Italian seasoning

1.

Preheat the oven to 375 degrees Fahrenheit.

2.

Using cooking spray, coat the baking dish.

3.

Combine mayonnaise, garlic powder, poultry spice, and pepper in a small bowl.

4.

Place the chicken breasts in the baking dish that has been prepared.

5.

Spread the mayonnaise mixture over the chicken, then top with cheese.

6.

For 35 minutes, bake the chicken.

7.

Serve and have fun.

Nutritional Value (Serving Size):

391 calories

Fat 23 g

11 g carbohydrates

Sugar 3 g

33 g protein

112 mg cholesterol

Chapter Ten

Chicken Wings

Time to prepare: 10 minutes

30 minutes to prepare

Serve: 6

Ingredients:

1 beaten egg

1/2 pound chicken wings

6 tablespoons olive oil

apple cider vinegar, 1/2 cup

1/2 teaspoon cayenne

2 minced garlic cloves

1 teaspoon pepper

3/4 teaspoon salt Instructions:

1.

In a large mixing basin, combine all ingredients except the chicken and stir thoroughly.

2.

In a mixing bowl, combine the chicken wings with the sauce and leave aside for 20 minutes.

3.

Preheat the oven to 450 degrees Fahrenheit.

4.

Using cooking spray, coat a baking tray.

5.

Bake the marinated wings for 30 minutes on a preheated baking tray.

6.

Serve and have fun.

Nutritional Value (Serving Size):

355 calories

Fat 23 g

0.5 g carbohydrates

Sugar 0.1 g

33 g protein

128 mg cholesterol

Chapter Eleven

Chicken with Lemon

Time to prepare: 10 minutes

45 minutes to prepare

Serve: 8

Ingredients:

8 skinless and boneless chicken breasts

1 tablespoon lemon juice

2 tablespoons chopped green onion

1 tablespoon oregano

3 oz. crumbled feta cheese

1/4 teaspoon pepper Instructions:

1.

Preheat the oven to 350 degrees Fahrenheit.

2.

Using cooking spray, coat the baking dish.

3.

Place the chicken breasts in the baking dish you've prepared.

4.

2 tablespoons lemon juice, 1/2 tablespoon oregano, and pepper

5.

Green onion and crumbled cheese go on top.

6.

Drizzle with oregano and the remaining lemon juice.

7.

45 minutes in the oven

8.

Serve and have fun.

Nutritional Value (Serving Size):

246 calories

Fat 10.8 g

1.2 g carbohydrates

Sugar 0.5 g

34 g protein

110 mg cholesterol

Chapter Twelve

Delicious Chicken Skewers

Time to prepare: 10 minutes

Serve: 8

Ingredients:

2 pound tenderloins of chicken breast

1 teaspoon salt and pepper

1 teaspoon minced garlic

1 tablespoon extra virgin olive oil

1 cup salsa Instructions:

1.

In a zip-lock bag, combine the chicken, 1/4 cup salsa, lemon pepper spice, garlic, and oil.

2.

Refrigerate the bag overnight after sealing it and shaking it firmly.

3.

Using moistened wooden skewers, thread marinated chicken onto them.

4.

Cook for 8-10 minutes on a hot grill with skewers.

5.

During the last 3 minutes of grilling, brush with the remaining salsa.

6.

Serve and have fun.

Nutritional Value (Serving Size):

125 calories

Fat 2.5 g

2.1 g carbohydrates

Sugar 1 g

24 g protein

71 mg cholesterol

Chapter Thirteen

Delicious Shredded Chicken

Time to prepare: 25 minutes

Serve: 6

Ingredients:

3 boneless and skinless chicken breasts

1 tablespoon of vinegar

chunky salsa (13.5 oz)

1 teaspoon onion powder

1 tablespoon cumin powder

1 1/2 tablespoons chilli powder

1.

In the instant pot, combine all ingredients and stir well.

2.

Cook on manual high pressure for 25 minutes after sealing the pot.

3.

After that, use the quick-release method to release pressure before opening the lid.

4.

Take the chicken out of the pot and shred it with a fork.

5.

Serve and have fun.

Nutritional Value (Serving Size):

171 calories

Fat 6.3 g

5 g carbohydrates

Sugar 2.2 g

23 g protein

64 mg cholesterol

Chapter Fourteen

Yogurt Chicken

15 minutes to prepare

Serve: 5

Ingredients:

2 pound skinless and boneless chicken breast

a half-cup of Greek yoghurt

1 tablespoon mayonnaise

1/2 teaspoon of herb seasoning

1/2 teaspoon of onion powder and 1/2 teaspoon of garlic powder

1/4 teaspoon salt Instructions:

1.

Preheat the air fryer to 380 degrees Fahrenheit.

2.

Combine mayonnaise, herb seasoning, onion powder, garlic powder, and yoghurt in a small bowl.

3.

Coat the chicken with the mayonnaise mixture.

4.

Using cooking spray, coat the air fryer basket.

5.

Cook the chicken for 15 minutes in an air fryer basket. Halfway through, turn around.

6.

Serve and have fun.

Nutritional Value (Serving Size):

272 calories

Fat 8 g

5 g carbohydrates

Sugar 2 g

40 g protein

121 mg cholesterol

Chapter Fifteen

Salad with Chicken Bacon

Time to prepare: 10 minutes

Serve: 4

Ingredients:

2 cooked and sliced chicken breasts

3 cooked and sliced bacon slices

1/2 cup diced celery

2 avocados, diced

2 1/2 tablespoons extra virgin olive oil

3 tablespoons lemon juice

1 teaspoon dried dill

1 tablespoon chives, dried

1 teaspoon pepper

1 teaspoon salt Instructions:

1.

Toss all of the ingredients together in a large mixing basin.

2.

Serve and have fun.

Nutritional Value (Serving Size):

441 calories

Fat 36 g

10 g carbohydrates

Sugar 1 g

24 g protein

66 mg cholesterol

Chapter Sixteen

Mahi Mahi grilled

Seafood

Time to prepare: 10 minutes

Serve: 6

Ingredients:

6 fillets of mahi-mahi

14 cup chicken stock 12 teaspoon minced garlic

1 minced little onion

6 tablespoons butter

2 tablespoons olive oil

2 tablespoons lemon juice Instructions:

1.

Preheat your grill to medium-high.

2.

Fill a mixing dish halfway with fish fillets. Coat the fish fillets thoroughly in oil, pepper, and salt.

3.

Cook the fish for 3-4 minutes on each side on a hot grill.

4.

Place the fish in a serving dish.

5.

1 tablespoon butter, melted in a skillet over medium-high heat

6.

Add the onion and cook for 2 minutes, or until softened.

7.

Sauté for a minute after adding the garlic.

8.

Simmer until the liquid has been reduced by half.

9.

Cook for a minute after adding the lemon juice.

10.

Remove the skillet from the heat and whisk in the remaining butter until the sauce thickens.

11.

Serve the sauce over the cooked fish.

Nutritional Value (Serving Size):

237 calories

Fat 16.2 g

1.2 g carbohydrates

Sugar 0.5 g

21.3 g protein

71 mg cholesterol

Chapter Seventeen

Salad with Crab

Time to prepare: 10 minutes

Time to prepare: 10 minutes

Serve: 6

Ingredients:

Crab meat, 8 ounces

2 cut celery stalks

12 teaspoon Worcestershire

12 teaspoon old bay seasoning

12 teaspoon dried dill

1 tablespoon lemon juice

2 tbsp chopped fresh parsley

1 tablespoon mayonnaise

sour cream (12 cup)

cream cheese, 4 ounce

1 teaspoon crushed garlic

14 cup diced onion

2 tablespoons of butter

1.

In a small saucepan over medium heat, melt the butter.

2.

Add the onion and cook until it is softened.

3.

Sauté for a minute after adding the garlic.

4.

Place the onion-garlic combination in a large mixing basin.

5.

Toss in the remaining ingredients and whisk thoroughly to incorporate.

6.

Serve and have fun.

Nutritional Value (Serving Size):

219 calories

Fat 18.4 g

5.6 g carbohydrates

Sugar 1.1 g

7.2 g protein

62 mg cholesterol

Chapter Eighteen

Shrimp with Garlic

Time to prepare: 10 minutes

Time to prepare: 10 minutes

Serve: 4

Ingredients:

1 pound shrimp

2 tbsp chopped fresh parsley

12 cup grated parmesan cheese

12 gallon heavy cream

12 cup stock (chicken)

5 minced garlic cloves

2 tablespoons butter

1 tablespoon extra virgin olive oil

Pepper

Salt

Directions:

1.

In a large skillet, heat the olive oil over medium-high heat.

2.

Season the shrimp with pepper and salt and cook for 1-2 minutes on each side in the pan.

3.

Place the shrimp in a basin and set aside.

4.

In the same pan, melt the butter. Sauté for a minute after adding the garlic.

5.

Cook until the stock has been reduced by half.

6.

Reduce the heat to low. Stir in the cream and cook for another 23 minutes.

7.

Cook, stirring constantly, until the cheese has melted.

8.

Return the shrimp to the skillet.

9.

Serve garnished with parsley.

Nutritional Value (Serving Size):

453 calories

Fat 32.4 g

4.5 g carbohydrates

Sugar 0.2 g

33.2 g protein

331 mg cholesterol

Chapter Nineteen

Salad de poisson facile

Time to prepare: 10 minutes

3 minute cooking time

Serve: 4

Ingredients:

8 ounces of shrimp

Crab meat, 8 ounces

1 tablespoon chopped dill

mayonnaise (12 cup)

2 teaspoons lemon juice

14 teaspoon of old bay seasoning

14 cup minced onion

12 cup chopped celery

1 quartered lemon

Pepper

Salt

Directions:

1.

Bring the lemon and water to a boil in the pot.

2.

Cook for 1-2 minutes after adding the shrimp to the saucepan.

3.

Drain the shrimp thoroughly and throw it in a large mixing dish.

4.

Stir in the other ingredients until thoroughly mixed.

5.

Refrigerate the salad bowl for 2 hours after covering it.

6.

Enjoy while it's still cold.

Nutritional Value (Serving Size):

240 calories

Fat 11 g

10 g carbohydrates

Sugar 2.4 g

20.6 g protein

157 mg cholesterol

Chapter Twenty

Crab Cakes Made Simple

Time to prepare: 10 minutes

Time to prepare: 10 minutes

Serve: 2

Ingredients:

Crab meat, 8 ounces

2 tablespoons butter

14 teaspoon pepper

12 teaspoon of old bay seasoning

1 tablespoon mayonnaise

1 gently beaten egg

a quarter cup of almond flour

14 cup chopped red pepper

1 tiny chopped onion Directions:

1.

In a mixing bowl, combine all ingredients except the butter and stir until well blended.

2.

From the bowl mixture, make tiny patties.

3.

In a medium saucepan, melt the butter.

4.

Cook crab cakes in batches for 2-3 minutes on each side, or until golden brown.

5.

Serve and have fun.

Nutritional Value (Serving Size):

311 calories

Fat 20.7 g

10.3 g carbohydrates

Sugar 3.4 g

17.8 g protein

177 mg cholesterol

Healthy Tuna Patties

Time to prepare: 10 minutes

15 minutes to prepare

Serve: 8

Ingredients:

2 drained and flaked tuna cans

4 tablespoons olive oil

14 cup chopped fresh parsley

2 lightly beaten eggs

3 minced garlic cloves

2 tablespoons mustard

1 tablespoon mayonnaise

14 teaspoon pepper

12 teaspoon salt Instructions:

1.

Preheat the oven to 170 degrees Fahrenheit.

2.

Combine tuna, parsley, eggs, garlic, Dijon mustard, mayonnaise, pepper, and salt in a mixing bowl.

3.

In a medium-sized skillet, heat the oil.

4.

Make tiny patties with the tuna mixture and fry for 2-3 minutes per side until golden brown.

5.

Serve and have fun.

Nutritional Value (Serving Size):

178 calories

Fat 13.1 g

1.7 g carbohydrates

Sugar 0.4 g

13.5 g protein

56 mg cholesterol

Chapter Twenty-one

Cod in Butter

Time to prepare: 10 minutes

Time to cook: 5 minutes

Serve: 4

Ingredients:

12 pound fillets of fish, sliced into pieces

12 teaspoon paprika

14 teaspoon pepper

1 tablespoon garlic powder

6 tablespoons butter

12 teaspoon salt Instructions:

1.

Combine paprika, pepper, garlic powder, and salt in a small bowl.

2.

Season the fish with the seasoning combination.

3.

In a large skillet, melt 2 tablespoons butter over medium-high heat.

4.

Cook for 2 minutes after adding the fish pieces to the pan.

5.

Reduce the heat to medium. Cook for 3-4 minutes with the remaining butter on top of the fish pieces.

6.

Remove the pan from the heat once the fish is fully done.

7.

Stir in the lemon juice thoroughly.

8.

Serve and have fun.

Nutritional Value (Serving Size):

291 calories

Fat 18.8 g

0.4 g carbohydrates

Sugar 0.1 g

30.6 g protein

129 mg cholesterol

Chapter Twenty-two

Tilapia Bake

Time to prepare: 10 minutes

Time to prepare: 10 minutes

Serve: 4

Ingredients:

4 fillets of tilapia

1 teaspoon lemon zest

2 tablespoons lemon juice

1 tablespoon minced garlic

14 cup melted butter

2 tbsp chopped fresh parsley

Pepper

Salt

Directions:

1.

Preheat the oven to 425 degrees Fahrenheit.

2.

Set aside a small bowl containing butter, lemon zest, lemon juice, and garlic.

3.

Season the fish fillets with salt and pepper.

4.

Fill the baking dish halfway with fish fillets. Brush the fish fillets with the butter mixture.

5.

Cook for 10-12 minutes in a preheated oven.

6.

Serve garnished with parsley.

Nutritional Value (Serving Size):

247 calories

Fat 13.6 g

1 g carbohydrate

Sugar 0.2 g

32.4 g protein

116 mg cholesterol

Chapter Twenty-three

Avocado Salad with Shrimp

Time to prepare: 10 minutes

Time to cook: 5 minutes

Serve: 4

Ingredients:

16 oz. thawed and drained shrimp

1 pitted and diced avocado

14 cup chopped celery

1 sliced tiny onion

2 12 tbsp chopped fresh dill

1 tablespoon of vinegar

1 teaspoon mustard

mayonnaise (12 cup)

Pepper

Salt

Directions:

1.

Combine mayonnaise, dill, vinegar, and mustard in a small bowl.

Place aside.

2.

In a mixing basin, combine the shrimp, onion, and celery.

3.

Stir the mayonnaise mixture into the shrimp.

4.

Refrigerate for 1-2 hours after covering with plastic wrap.

5.

Serve immediately with avocado.

Nutritional Value (Serving Size):

279 calories

Fat 13.1 g

12.5 g carbohydrates

Sugar 2.7 g

27 g protein

246 mg cholesterol

Chapter Twenty-four

Shrimp with Paprika

Time to prepare: 10 minutes

Time to prepare: 50 minutes

Serve: 8

Ingredients:

2 pound peeled and deveined shrimp

1 tablespoon paprika

5 chopped garlic cloves

3/4 cup extra virgin olive oil

1/2 teaspoon crushed red pepper flakes

1 teaspoon pepper

1 teaspoon of kosher salt

1.

Stir together the oil, red pepper flakes, pepper, paprika, garlic, and salt in the slow cooker.

2.

Cook for 30 minutes on high, covered.

3.

Serve with shrimp. Cook for 10 minutes, stirring occasionally.

4.

Cover and cook for another 10 minutes.

5.

Serve and have fun.

Nutritional Value (Serving Size):

300 calories

Fat 20.2 g

2.7 g carbohydrates

Sugar 0.3 g

25 g protein

240 mg cholesterol

Chapter Twenty-five

Soups and Side Dishes

Asparagus Soup with Cream

Time to prepare: 10 minutes

15 minutes to prepare

Serve: 6

Ingredients:

2 pound asparagus, cut ends off and chop into 12-inch segments

2 tablespoons olive oil

3 minced garlic cloves

2 ounces grated parmesan cheese

12 gallon heavy cream

14 cup chopped onion

4 c. vegetable broth

Pepper

Salt

Directions:

1.

In a large pot, heat the olive oil over medium heat.

2.

Add the onion to the pot and cook until softened.

3.

Sauté the asparagus for 2-3 minutes.

4.

Sauté for a minute after adding the garlic. Season with salt and pepper.

5.

Bring the stock to a boil. Reduce the heat to low and continue to cook until the asparagus is tender.

6.

Remove the soup from the heat and purée it with an immersion blender until smooth.

7.

Return the pot to the heat. Cook over medium heat, stirring constantly, until the soup is just heated. The soup should not be cooked.

8.

Turn off the heat. Stir in the cheese thoroughly.

9.

Serve and have fun.

Nutritional Value (Serving Size):

146 calories

Fat 11.9 g

8.8 g carbohydrates

Sugar 4.4 g

6.7 g protein

20 mg cholesterol

Chapter Twenty-six

Soup with Celery

Time to prepare: 10 minutes

Time to prepare: 20 minutes

Serve: 4

Ingredients:

3 cups chopped celery

1 quart vegetable stock

cream cheese, 5 ounce

12 tbsp chopped fresh basil

14 cup chopped onion 1 tablespoon chopped garlic

1 tablespoon extra virgin olive oil

14 teaspoon pepper

12 teaspoon salt Instructions:

1.

In a large saucepan, heat the oil over medium heat.

2.

In a saucepan, sauté the onion, garlic, and celery for 4-5 minutes, or until softened.

3.

Bring the broth to a boil. Reduce the heat to low and continue to cook.

4.

Stir in the basil and cream cheese until the cheese has melted.

5.

Season the soup with salt and pepper.

6.

Remove the soup from the heat and purée it with an immersion blender until it is smooth and creamy.

7.

Serve and have fun.

Nutritional Value (Serving Size):

182 calories

Fat 16.4 g

4.9 g carbohydrates

Sugar 1.6 g

4.7 g protein

39 mg cholesterol

Chapter Twenty-seven

Soup with Cauliflower Flavor

Time to prepare: 10 minutes

Time to prepare: 25 minutes

Serve: 6

Ingredients:

3 cups florets de cauliflower

12 cup heavy cream 3.5 ounces cream cheese

3 c. vegetable broth

12 tbsp chopped fresh thyme

1 tablespoon minced garlic

2 tablespoons olive oil

2 tablespoons butter

14 teaspoon pepper

14 teaspoon salt Instructions:

1.

Preheat the oven to 425 degrees Fahrenheit.

2.

Drizzle oil over the cauliflower florets on the baking tray. Season with salt and pepper.

3.

Set aside after roasting cauliflower in a preheated oven for 10-15 minutes.

4.

In a large pot over medium heat, melt the butter.

5.

Sauté for a minute with the thyme and garlic.

6.

Stir in the cream, cream cheese, and stock. Cook, stirring occasionally, until the cheese has melted.

7.

Bring to a boil with the roasted cauliflower. Reduce the heat to low and cook for 10 minutes.

8.

Remove the soup from the heat and mix it with an immersion blender until smooth.

9.

Serve and have fun.

Nutritional Value (Serving Size):

187 calories

Fat 19.1 g

5 g carbohydrates

Sugar 2.3 g

2.6 g protein

42 mg cholesterol

Chapter Twenty-eight

Zucchini Basil Soup

Time to prepare: 10 minutes

Time to prepare: 25 minutes

Serve: 4

Ingredients:

2 chopped medium zucchinis

14 cup basil leaves, fresh

3 quarts vegetable stock

3 tablespoons olive oil

1 tablespoon minced garlic

1 medium sliced onion

14 teaspoon pepper

12 teaspoon salt Instructions:

1.

In a medium saucepan, heat the olive oil.

2.

Sauté the garlic and onion for 3-5 minutes, or until the onion has softened.

3.

Cook for 5 minutes after adding the zucchini.

4.

Bring the stock to a boil. Reduce the heat to low and cook for 15 minutes.

5.

Turn off the heat. Stir in the basil well.

6.

Using an immersion blender, puree the soup until it is completely smooth.

7.

Season the soup with salt and pepper.

8.

Serve and have fun.

Nutritional Value (Serving Size):

149 calories

Fat 11.8 g

7.3 g carbohydrates

Sugar 3.4 g

5.3 g protein

Chapter Twenty-nine

Chicken Soup, Warm and Delicious

Time to prepare: 10 minutes

Time to prepare: 20 minutes

Serve: 4

Ingredients:

4 skinless, deboned, cooked, and chopped chicken thighs

2 tbsp chopped fresh parsley

2 chopped celery ribs

3 c. chicken broth

12 gallon heavy cream

12 c. coconut milk

1/3 cup liquid

3 ounces sliced mushrooms

1 tablespoon minced garlic

2 tablespoons butter

3 cooked and sliced bacon slices

Pepper

Salt

Directions:

1.

In a large pot over medium heat, melt the butter.

2.

Cook until the mushrooms have softened, then add the garlic.

3.

Cook until the water has been reduced by half.

4.

Combine the stock, heavy cream, and coconut milk in a mixing bowl.

5.

Combine the chicken and celery. Stir thoroughly and cook until the soup is just hot.

The soup should not be cooked.

6.

Season the soup with salt and pepper.

7.

Serve with bacon and parsley on top.

8.

Serve and have fun.

Nutritional Value (Serving Size):

543 calories

Fat 35.8 g

4.6 g carbohydrates

Sugar 2.1 g

50 g protein

181 mg cholesterol

Chapter Thirty

Soup with Creamy Mushrooms

Time to prepare: 10 minutes

Time to cook: 40 minutes

Serve: 4

Ingredients:

1 pound cleaned and sliced mushroom

12 gallon heavy cream

12 teaspoon dried thyme

4 c. vegetable broth

3 tablespoons butter

14 cup chopped onion

Pepper

Salt

Directions:

1.

In a large pot over medium heat, melt the butter.

2.

Add the onion and cook for another 2-3 minutes.

3.

Cook for 4-5 minutes after adding the mushrooms.

4.

Stir in the thyme and stock well. Simmer for 30 minutes with the cover on the pot.

5.

Remove the soup from the heat and purée it in a blender until smooth.

6.

Stir in the heavy cream well. Season the soup with salt and pepper.

7.

Serve and have fun.

Nutritional Value (Serving Size):

158 calories

Fat 15 g

5.4 g carbohydrates

Sugar 2.8 g

4.1 g protein

43 mg cholesterol

Chapter Thirty-one

Soup with Kale and Cauliflower

Time to prepare: 10 minutes

1 hour and 20 minutes of cooking

Serve: 4

Ingredients:

4 cups florets de cauliflower

6 c. vegetable broth

1 tablespoon minced garlic

14 cup chopped onion

6 oz. chopped kale

6 tablespoons olive oil

Pepper

Salt

Directions:

1.

Preheat the oven to 425 degrees Fahrenheit.

2.

Pour 2 tablespoons of oil over the cauliflower on the baking dish and season with pepper and salt.

3.

Roast cauliflower for 25 minutes in a preheated oven. Take it out of the oven and set it aside.

4.

Toss kale with 2 tablespoons oil and salt in a mixing basin.

Arrange the kale on the baking tray and bake for 30 minutes at 300 degrees F. Halfway through, toss.

5.

In a large saucepan over medium heat, heat the remaining oil.

6.

Sauté the onion for 3-4 minutes. Sauté for a minute after adding the garlic.

7.

Bring the stock and roasted cauliflower to a boil.

8.

Reduce the heat to low and cook for 10 minutes.

9.

Cook for another 10 minutes with the kale.

10.

Remove the soup from the heat and purée it with an immersion blender until smooth.

11.

Serve and have fun.

Nutritional Value (Serving Size):

235 calories

Fat 21.6 g

11.6 g carbohydrates

Sugar 3.2 g

3.5 g protein

0 mg cholesterol

Chapter Thirty-two

Pumpkin Soup

Time to prepare: 10 minutes

15 minutes to prepare

Serve: 6

Ingredients:

14.5 ounces pureed pumpkin

12 gallon heavy cream

2 tbsp chopped fresh parsley

12 teaspoon thyme, chopped

12 tablespoons garlic powder

4 c. vegetable broth

14 teaspoon pepper

12 teaspoon salt Instructions:

1.

Stir together all of the ingredients in the saucepan, except the heavy cream. Over medium-high heat, bring to a boil.

2.

Reduce the heat to low and cook for 10 minutes.

3.

Turn off the heat. Stir in the heavy cream well.

4.

Serve garnished with parsley.

Nutritional Value (Serving Size):

61 calories

Fat 4.2 g

6.4 g carbohydrates

Sugar 2.7 g

1 g protein

14 mg cholesterol

Chapter Thirty-three

Cauliflower Soup with Chicken

Time to prepare: 10 minutes

Time to prepare: 10 minutes

Serve: 4

Ingredients:

2 cups cooked and shredded chicken

4 oz. cubed cream cheese

1 tablespoon minced garlic

2 tablespoons butter

12 cup cooked cauliflower rice

12 teaspoon powdered onion

14 gallon heavy cream

Salt 14.5 ounces chicken stock

Directions:

1.

In a medium saucepan over medium heat, melt the butter.

2.

Sauté for a minute after adding the garlic. Stir in the chicken well.

3.

Stir in the cream cheese until it is completely melted.

4.

Stock, onion powder, heavy cream, and salt are added to the pot. Bring to a boil over medium-high heat, stirring constantly.

5.

Reduce the heat to low and cook for 3-4 minutes.

6.

Cook for 2-3 minutes after adding the cauliflower rice.

7.

Serve and have fun.

Nutritional Value (Serving Size):

299 calories

Fat 20.8 g

4.2 g carbohydrates

Sugar 1.4 g

23.8 g protein

111 mg cholesterol

Chapter Thirty-four

Cauliflower Soup with Chicken

Time to prepare: 10 minutes

Time to prepare: 10 minutes

Serve: 6

Ingredients:

1 large head of cauliflower, florets

1 tablespoon chopped fresh parsley

14 teaspoon paprika

1 tablespoon onion powder

2 tablespoons butter

1/3 cup cream de coco

Pepper

Salt

Directions:

1.

In a microwave-safe bowl, combine cauliflower florets and 2 tablespoons water. Microwave for 5 minutes, covered.

2.

Microwave for another 5 minutes after stirring the cauliflower.

3.

Place the cauliflower in a food processor and drain well. Process the remaining ingredients, except the parsley, until smooth and creamy.

4.

Serve garnished with parsley.

Nutritional Value (Serving Size):

102 calories

Fat 7.2 g

8.6 g carbohydrates

Sugar 4 g

3.2 g protein

10 mg cholesterol

Chapter Thirty-five

Desserts

Mug Cake

Time to prepare: 5 minutes

2 minute cooking time

Serve: 1

Ingredients:

1 gently beaten egg

1/8 teaspoon gluten-free baking powder

2 tbsp peanut butter (creamy)

1 tablespoon of Swerve

1.

In a microwave-safe mug, combine all ingredients and stir until well incorporated.

2.

Microwave for 1-2 minutes in a microwave-safe cup.

3.

Serve and have fun.

Nutritional Value (Serving Size):

257 calories

Fat 20.5 g

8.9 g carbohydrates

Sugar 3.3 g

13.5 g protein

164 mg cholesterol

Chapter Thirty-six

Fat Bombs Chocó

Time to prepare: 10 minutes

Time to cook: 5 minutes

Serve: 30

Ingredients:

3.5 ounces dark chocolate, unsweetened

6 drops stevia liquid

14 cup coconut oil Instructions:

1.

Microwave the chocolate, oil, and sweetener in a microwave-safe bowl until the chocolate is completely melted.

2.

Place the mould in the refrigerator until the chocolate mixture has firm.

3.

Serve and have fun.

Nutritional Value (Serving Size):

38 calories

Fat 3.6 g

0.9 g carbohydrates

Sugar 0 g

0.4 g protein

0 mg cholesterol

Chapter Thirty-seven

Frosty Chocolate Delight

Time to prepare: 10 minutes

Time to prepare: 10 minutes

Serve: 2

Ingredients:

12 cup heavy cream (whipped)

12 tablespoons lakanto monk fruit

1 teaspoon vanilla

2 tbsp cocoa powder (unsweetened)

Directions:

1. In a large mixing basin, combine all of the ingredients.

2. Using a hand mixer, beat until peaks form.

3. Place the mixture in a zip-lock bag in the refrigerator for 45 minutes.

4. Take a zip-lock bag from the fridge and snip one of the corners.

5. Pour icy into serving dishes. Chill before serving.

Nutritional Value (Serving Size):

342 calories

Fat 34 g

6.3 g carbohydrates

Sugar 1 g

2.9 g protein

123 mg cholesterol

Chapter Thirty-eight

Mousse de strawberries

Time to prepare: 10 minutes

Time to cook: 5 minutes

Serve: 4

Ingredients:

1 cup heavy cream (whipped)

1 cup chopped fresh strawberries

2 tablespoons Swerve

1 pound of cream cheese Directions:

1. In a large mixing basin, whisk heavy whipping cream with a hand mixer until thickened.
2. Mix in the sweetener and cream cheese thoroughly.
3. Fold in the strawberries thoroughly.

4. Pour the mixture into serving glasses and chill for 1-2 hours.

5. Enjoy while chilled.

Nutritional Value (Serving Size):

320 calories

Fat 31.4 g

6.2 g carbohydrates

Sugar 1.9 g

5.2 g protein

105 mg cholesterol

Chapter Thirty-nine

Mousse Cheesecake

Time to prepare: 10 minutes

Time to cook: 5 minutes

Serve: 6

Ingredients:

1 cup heavy cream (whipped)

1 teaspoon vanilla extract

erythritol (14 cup)

8 ounces softened cream cheese Directions:

1. In a mixing bowl, whip the cream cheese until smooth.

2. Combine the vanilla and sweetener in a mixing bowl.

3. In a separate dish, whisk heavy cream until firm peaks form.

4. Fold the whipped cream into the cream cheese mixture and whisk until frothy with a hand mixer. Refrigerate for at least 2 hours.

5. Pipe into cold serving glasses and serve.

Nutritional Value (Serving Size):

203 calories

Fat 20.6 g

11.7 g carbohydrates

Sugar 10.2 g

3.3 g protein

69 mg cholesterol

Chapter Forty

Dessert with berries and cheese

Time to prepare: 10 minutes

Time to prepare: 10 minutes

Serve: 8

Ingredients:

1 12 pound ricotta

1 pound of blackberries

1 blueberry cup

1 pound of raspberries

12 teaspoon vanilla

erythritol (12 cup)

1 teaspoon of lemon zest

14 gallon heavy cream Directions:

1. In a mixing basin, whisk the ricotta, vanilla, sweetener, and heavy cream with a hand mixer until smooth.

2. Alternate layers of ricotta mixture with 14 cup berries in four serving cups.

3. Plate and serve.

Nutritional Value (Serving Size):

201 calories

Fat 12 g

9 g carbohydrates

Sugar 4 g

10 g protein

32 mg cholesterol

Chapter Forty-one

Fudge with Chocó Peanut Butter

Time to prepare: 10 minutes

Time to prepare: 10 minutes

Serve: 16

Ingredients:

12 pound of peanut butter

12 teaspoon vanilla

Swerve (14 cup)

2 12 tbsp chocolate powder, unsweetened

14 cup ghee Method:

1. Prepare a small baking dish by lining it with parchment paper and setting it aside.

2. Microwave the ghee and peanut butter in a microwave-safe basin until the ghee and peanut butter are melted.

3. Stir in the remaining ingredients and pour into the prepared baking dish.

4. Refrigerate for 1 hour or until completely firm.

5. Serve by cutting into pieces.

Nutritional Value (Serving Size):

78 calories

Fat 7.4 g

2.1 g carbohydrates

Sugar 0.8 g

2.2 g protein

8 mg cholesterol

Chapter Forty-two

Fat Bombs with Raspberry

Time to prepare: 5 minutes

Time to cook: 5 minutes

Serve: 8

Ingredients:

12 cup raspberries, fresh

3 tablespoons Swerve

2 tbsp melted coconut oil

8 ounces softened cream cheese Directions:

1. In a food processor, combine all ingredients and pulse until smooth.

2. Fill the small muffin mould halfway with the fat bomb mixture and chill for 45 minutes.

3. Plate and serve.

Nutritional Value (Serving Size):

134 calories

Fat 13.3 g

2.4 g carbohydrates

Sugar 0.4 g

2.2 g protein

31 mg cholesterol

Chapter Forty-three

Lemon Mug Cake in a Hurry

Time to prepare: 5 minutes

2 minute cooking time

Serve: 1

Ingredients:

12 teaspoon lemon rind 1 egg, lightly beaten

1 tablespoon melted butter

12 tablespoons lemon juice

2 tablespoons erythritol

14 tsp gluten-free baking powder

a quarter cup of almond flour Directions:

1. Combine almond flour, baking powder, and sweetener in a small mixing dish.

2. Whisk together the egg, lemon juice, and melted butter in the almond flour mixture.

3. Microwave the cake mixture for 90 seconds in a microwave-safe cup.

4. Plate and serve.

Nutritional Value (Serving Size):

385 calories

Fat 32 g

8 g carbohydrates

Sugar 1 g

13 g protein

195 mg cholesterol

Chapter Forty-four

Tiramisu Mousse, Smooth and Silky

Time to prepare: 5 minutes

Time to cook: 5 minutes

Serve: 2

Ingredients:

mascarpone cheese (12 cup)

1 tablespoon of erythritol

1 teaspoon cocoa powder, unsweetened Directions:

1. In a blender, combine all ingredients and blend until smooth.

2. Fill a piping bag halfway with the combined mixture and pipe into serving glasses.

3. Set aside for 1 hour in the refrigerator.

4. Enjoy while cooled.

Nutritional Value (Serving Size):

110 calories

Fat 8.2 g

2.4 g carbohydrates

Sugar 0.2 g

7.2 g protein

32 mg cholesterol

Chapter Forty-five

Conclusion

This book will show you how to modify the keto diet after 50 and for beginners, and what the diet's health benefits are. My purpose is to present you with all relevant information regarding the keto diet after 50.

This book contains many simple keto recipes that are both delicious and healthful.

CPSIA information can be obtained
at www.ICGtesting.com
Printed in the USA
LVHW061454240722
724256LV00012B/304